The ancient secrets prepper's guide: Healing properties of wild herbs & greens

By Demetra Gerontakis

Disclaimer

I am not a medical professional, nor a doctor. Using remedies is a personal decision. The information herein is offered for informational purposes solely, and is universal as so.

Nothing written within this book is approved by the FDA or intended to diagnose, treat, or prevent disease. Always seek medical advice by your health care practioner before using herbs that you are not familiar with as many of them can interact with medications or cause allergies and some others are a danger to pregnant or lactating woman.

The information in this book is for educational purposes only. The reader is responsible for his or her own actions and the author does not accept any responibilities for any liabilities or damages,real or perceived,resulting from the use of this information.

Herbs, spices, nuts, berries and wild greens have been widely used in the past. The earliest records are dated from the sixteenth century BC. And those are a compilation of works from previous centuries. The ancient Greeks, Egyptians, Mesopotamians are only few of the civilizations who used herbs in healing and preserving in the ancient world. After Alexander the great died in 323, Ptolemy Soter founded the Alexandrian library in which he uncovered hundreds of papyrus on which medicinal recipes were written. They had been collected from the countries in which Alexander had passed through during his conquest and thus we know through accumulated knowledge on text that the five greatest civilizations to use herbs in those times were ancient Greece, Egypt, Mesopotamia, Rome and India. In addition, it is also well known that in Minoan Crete, from reading cuneiform text we conclude that the Minoans used herbs such as saffron, dittany, rosemary and a plethora of other herbs as early as 2000 BC which are still widely used today thus we can understand the almost centurial ages as well as the best health world wide of those who live on the island of Crete. This small accumulation of herbs and wild greens is only a small part of a very vast variety of health boosters. It provides what each herb does for the human body and because they all have medicinal uses, they should always be taken with caution and many with the supervision of a health practitioner as they can interact with some medications. Always get an expert's advice.

Preppers should be prepared. Here are some of the most important foods one can find when in an emergency situation that will definitely prove potent and keep you and your family members alive during a season of tumoil.

The herbs within these pages can be made into tea, thrown on salads, used in medicinal creams and lotions, insect repellent sprays, essential oils, body rubs and much much more. It is everyones's duty to recognise and have the knowledge to use them instead of being dependent on pharmacies, governments etc.

Following ancient civilizations can prove to be a life saving experience.

Nettle: Urtica dioica is a leafy green.

Healing properties:

- seasonal allergies
- iron deficiency
- antibacterial
- anti inflammatory
- antioxidant
- anti rheumatism
- slows down early ageing
- cleanses toxins away
- hemorrhoids
- eczema
- uric acid

Vitamins & minerals: calcium, potassium, iron, B complex, K and C.

Can be used as a tea or eaten boiled lightly.

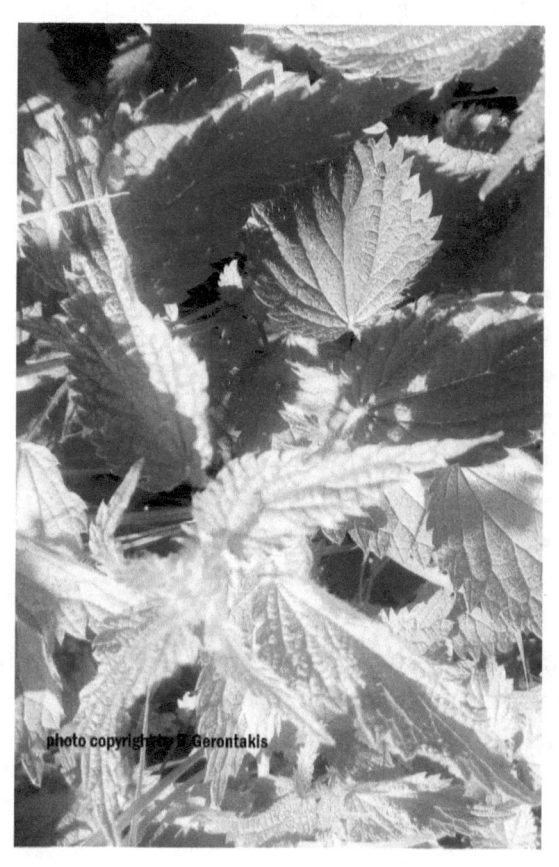

photo copyright by S. Gerontakis

Wild blackberry: Rubus – is a super food.

Healing properties:

- protects eyes
- lowers cholesterol
- arthritis
- weight control
- lowers blood pressure
- promotes a healthy heart
- lowers uric acid
- helps with kidney problems
- stop bleeding gums
- stops the development of some cancer cells.

Vitamins & minerals: C, A, E, folic acid, calcium, selenium, magnesium, phosphorus, potassium, zinc, protein and fiber.

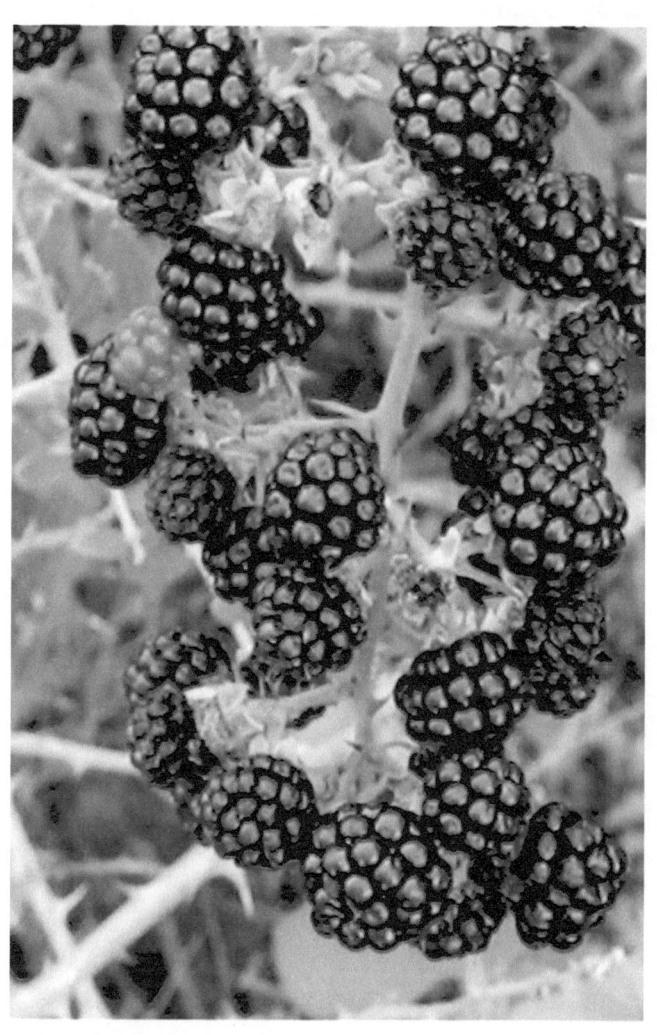

Zochos : Sochus Oleraceus – is a leafy green.

Healing properties:

- promotes a healthy heart
- constipation
- helps with liver problems
- insomnia
- restlessness
- nervous system
- hypersensitivity in children
- rheumatism
- muscle pain
- cough
- tranquillizer

Can be eaten raw in salads, boiled with olive oil and lemon juice and its juice can be consumed like a tea.

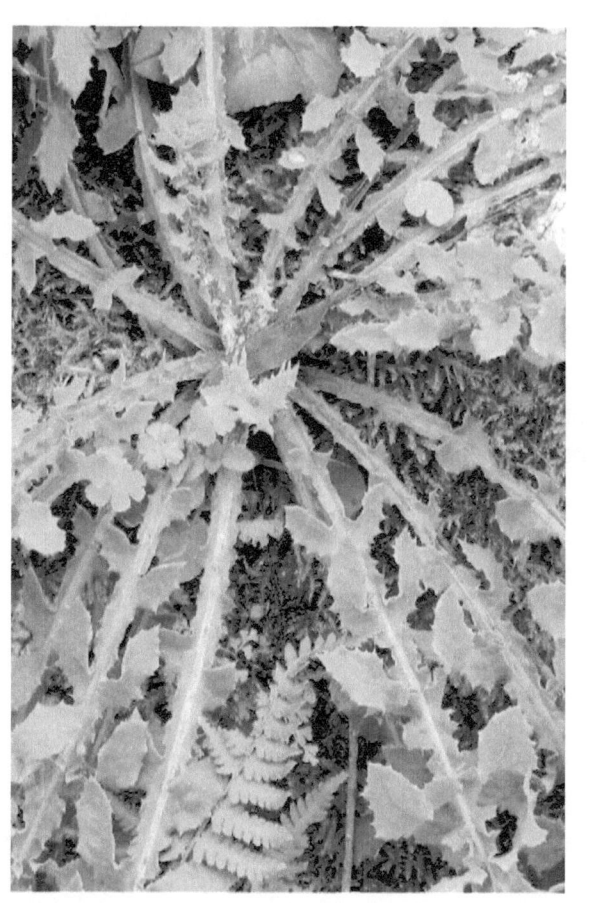

Red clover: Trifolium pretense – a green.

Healing properties:

- bronchitis
- menopause symptoms
- diuretic
- anti spasm
- anti cancer
- osteoporosis
- eczema
- breast cancer

Precautions:

Safe when taken in small amounts.

Do not take during pregnancy- consult your doctor.

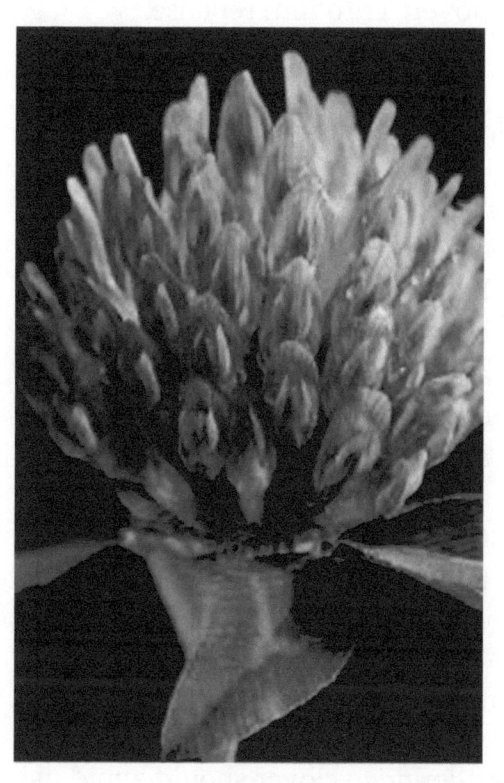

White clover: Trifolium repense

Healing properties:

- cleanses toxins from blood
- helps insomnia
- boosts appetite
- anti rheumatic/ rheumatism
- eye wash
- antiseptic
- arthritis
- flower beds used as a cleanser
- tea is used for fevers, colds and coughs

Precautions:

People allergic to clover should avoid using it.

If under medications for blood clots or hypertension avoid using clover as it has blood thinning properties.

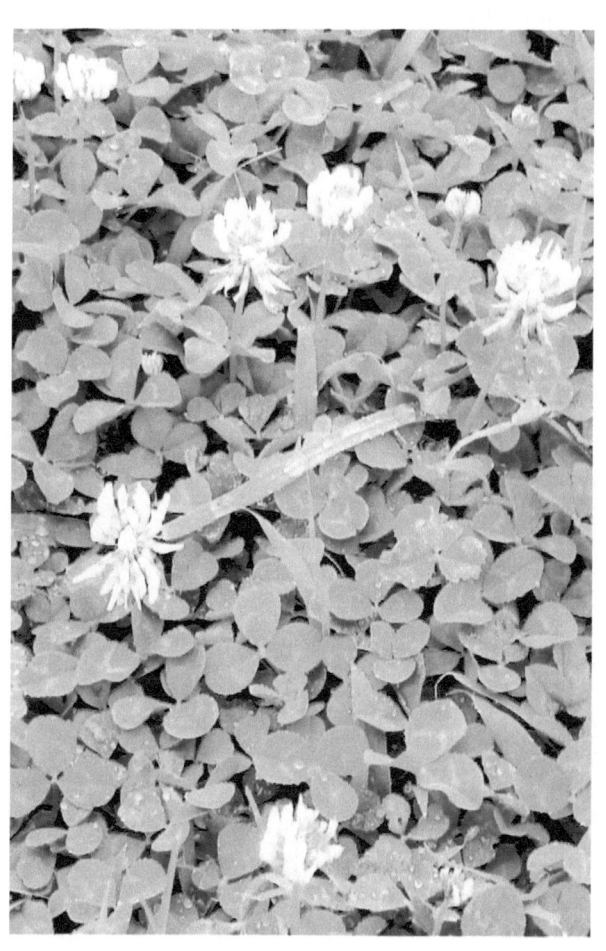

Common mallow: Malva sylvestris

Healing properties

- sore throat
- diuretic
- bronchitis
- cystitis
- intestinal disturbances
- cleanses toxins
- cleanses kidneys and liver
- hemorrhoids
- relieves water retention
- skin problems
- relieves swollen feet
- light burns

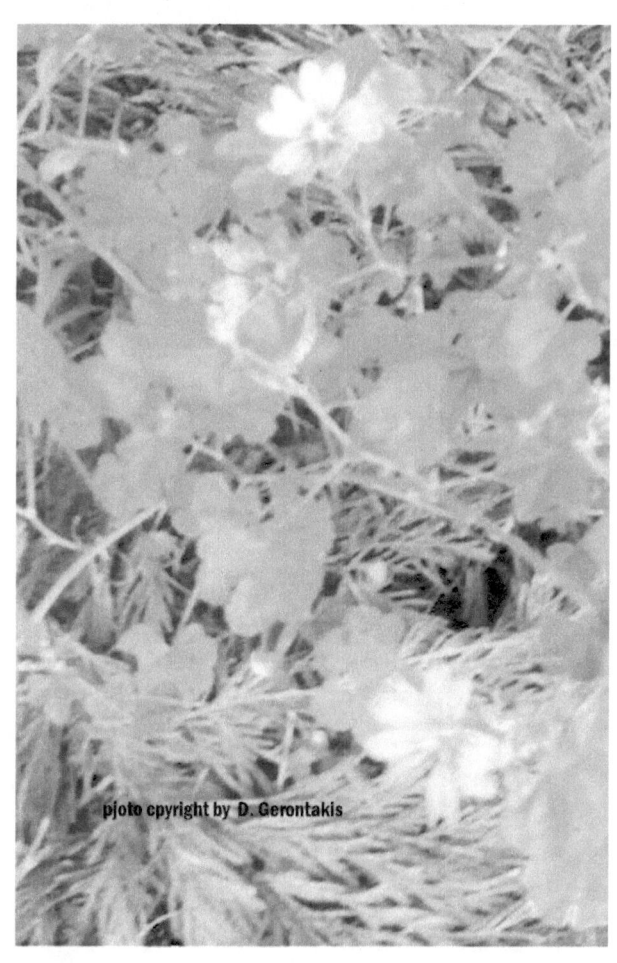

pjoto cpyright by D. Gerontakis

Wild dandelion: Taraxacum Officinale
Healing properties:

- diuretic
- boosts healthy blood flow for a healthy heart
- uric acid
- helps water retention before and during menstrual cycle
- helps hypertension
- anti scurvy
- stimulant
- anti flammatory
- lowers cholesterol as it adjusts triglycerides in the blood
- detoxifies every part of the body inside and out
- detoxifies and stimulates liver to work well
- helps cognitive function
- Cleanses gall bladder of toxins and supports
- Boosts calcium absorption
- Cleanses kidneys
- Excellent therapeutic for chronic dermatitis
- Controls constipation
- Boosts digestion
- Weight regulator
- Clears eczema

- Acne
- Rash
- Herpe virus
- Controls blood sugar and thus helps diabetes
- Cleanses the spleen from toxins
- Regulates glands
- Anti rheumatism
- Arthritis

Contains: carbohydrates, fiber, proteins, iron, best source of potassium,magnesium,manganese,sulfar,sodium ,zinc, flavonoids glycosides and vitamins A, C, D,E,K, B3,B2,B1 and Folic acid.

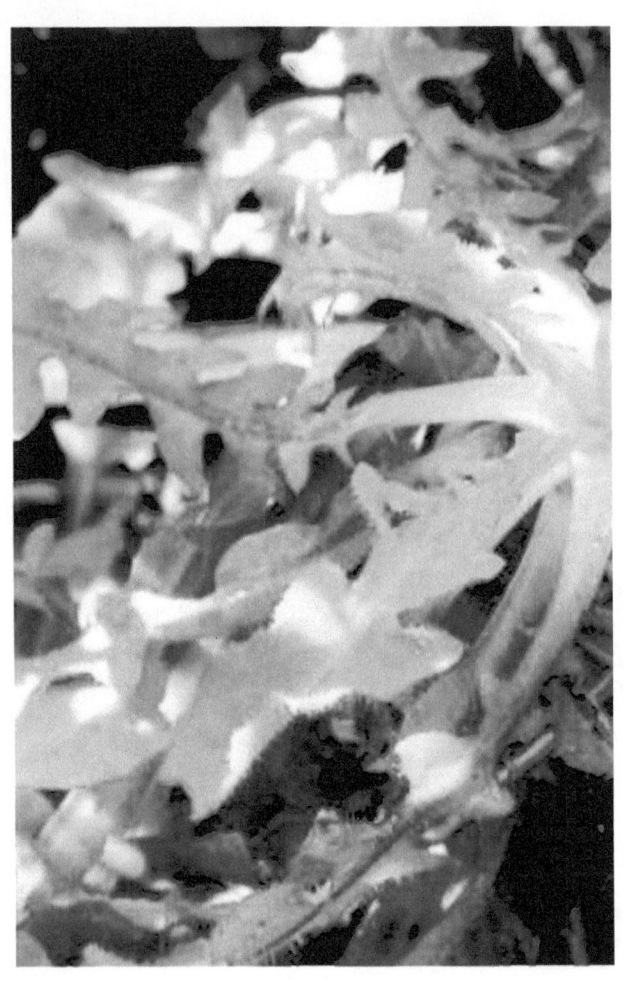

Marjoram: Origanum majorana (related to Oregano

Healing properties:

- insomnia
- migraines
- vertigo
- epilepsy
- loss of memory
- anti diabetes
- protects from stomach problems
- muscle pains
- antiseptic
- cough
- tonsillitis
- bronchitis
- reverses nausea
- anti spasm
- antioxidant
- mouth sores
- ear aches
- sinus
- flu
- rheumatism
- indigestion
- stimulates immune system
- measles
- salmonella

- malaria
- typhus
- polycystic syndrome

One of the most powerful antioxidant herbs next to oregano, thyme, lavender and rosemary.

Use in moderation in small quantities

Vitamin C, niacin, B6, A, folic acid. Beta carotene and fiber.

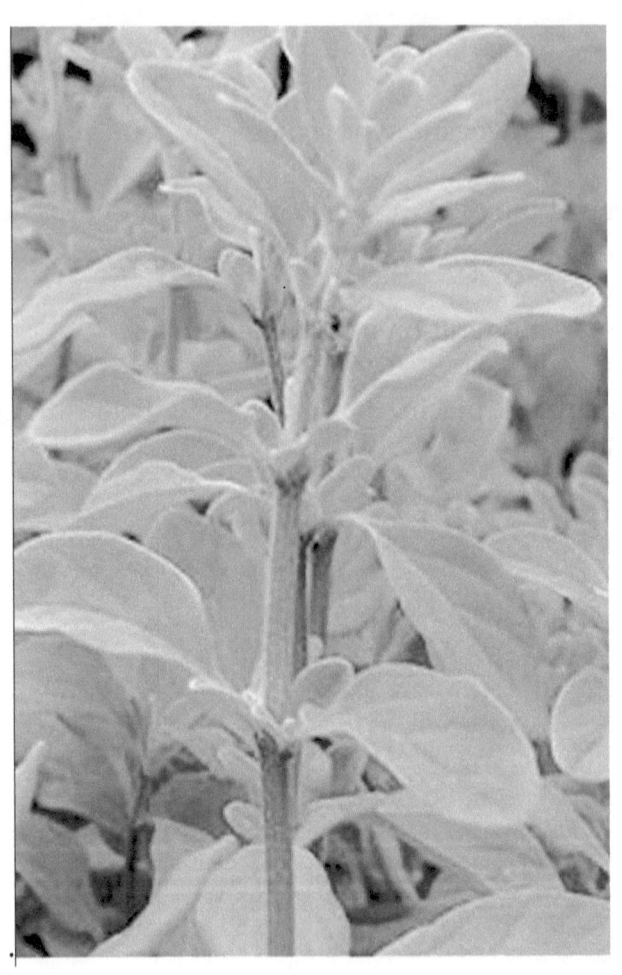

Oregano: Origanum Vulgare
Healing properties:

- toothache
- asthma and cough
- diarrhea
- rheumatism
- aids digestion
- heals wounds
- anti cough
- antioxidant
- antiseptic
- anti flammatory
- antibacterial
- anti cancerous
- analgesic indigestion
- herpes
- allergies
- sore throat
- arthritis
- bad breath
- stimulant for anemia
- Crohn's disease
- Dange fever
- earache
- Prostate and urinary tract infection
- Eczema
- Insect bites
- Gum disease

Is loaded with great amounts of vitamin C

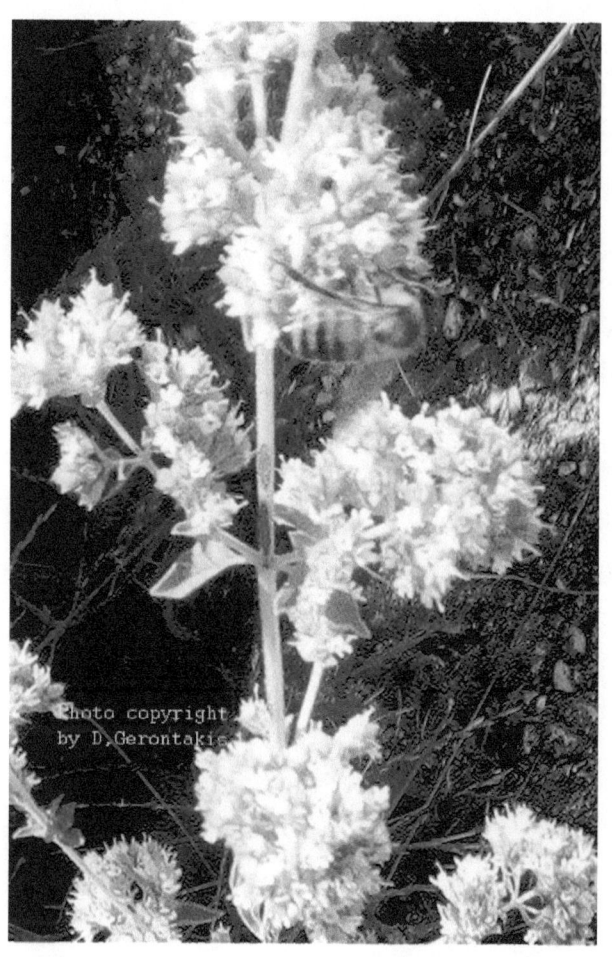

Thymus(thyme) vulgaris

Healing properties:

- cough
- respiratory problems
- diarrhea
- indigestion
- stomach ache
- insomnia
- streghtens skin
- stimulates and shines hair
- effective agaist acne
- acts against oily skin
- combats cellulite

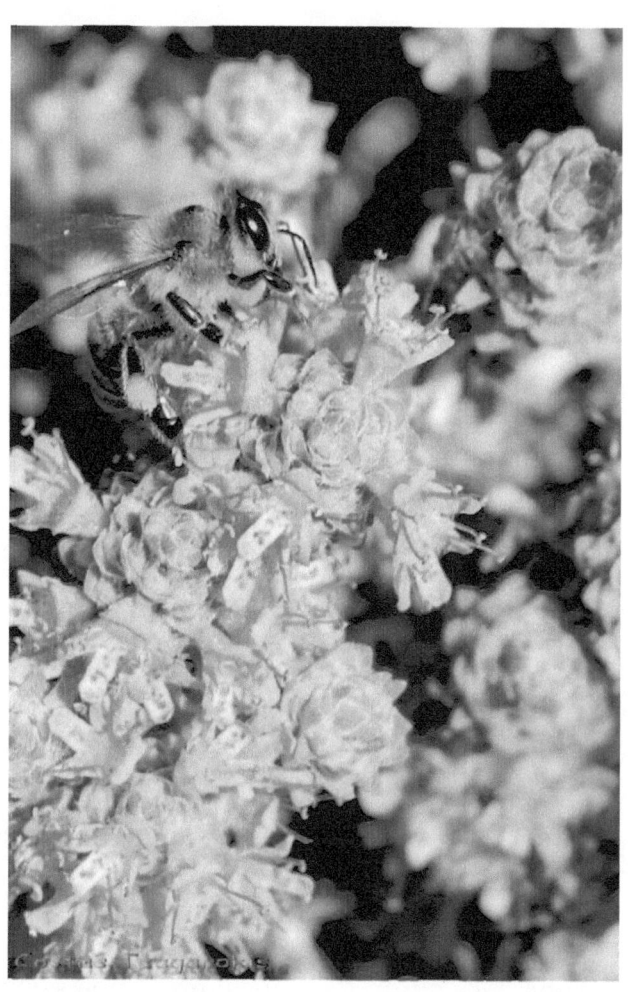

Chamomile: Asteraceae

Healing properties:

- calms nerves, enhances sleep
- helps insomnia,anti stress
- migraines,vertigo
- anxiety
- healing properties on cuts, bruises
- eczema
- anti flammatory
- skin & eye inflammations and infections
- gum disease and gingivitis
- stimulates immune system
- cold & flu
- anti spasm,antiseptic
- anti fever
- helps allergies
- menstrual cramps
- teething
- gas healing properties
- helps black circles around eyes

Contains: calcium, magnesium, potassium, fluoride, folate and vitamin A

No more than three cups a day for adults. Consult your doctor for children and young adults.

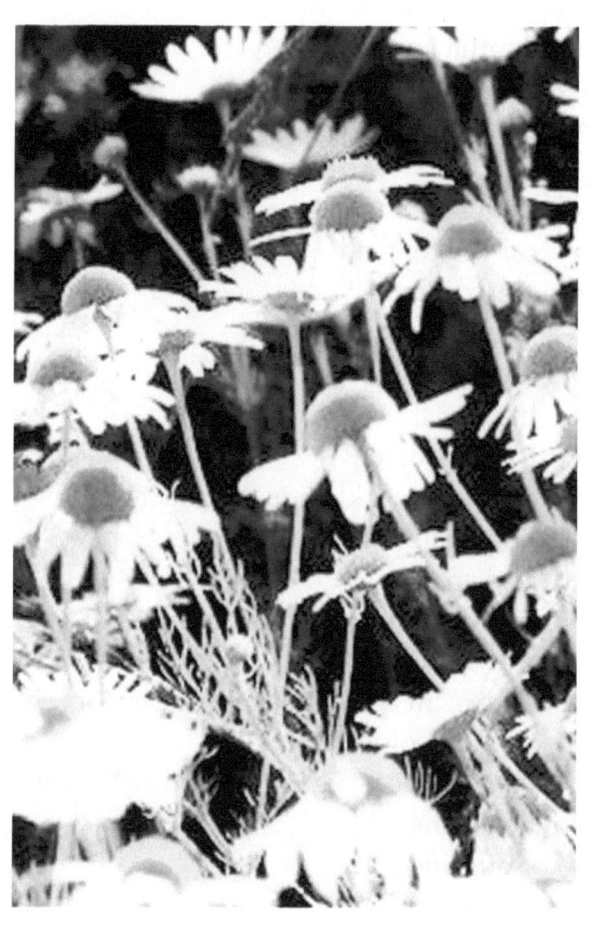

Mint: Mentha spicate

Healing properties:

- cleanses blood
- calms stomach
- antioxidant
- Crohn's disease
- diarrhea
- muscle cramps
- toxic virusus
- cleanses blackheads (antibacterial)
- helps memory
- anti spasm
- protects and recovers damages of DNA from radiation
- opens air passages in respiratory issues such as colds or flu
- protects body against creating cancer cells
- headaches
- sinus and allergies
- asthma
- mint is used to protect cancer patients' bodies who are subject to radiation
- polycystic syndrome

There are over twenty six different species of mint only in Greece.

Mint provides vitamin A,C, B12, B3, folic acid, magnesium, iron, calcium, potassium and manganese.

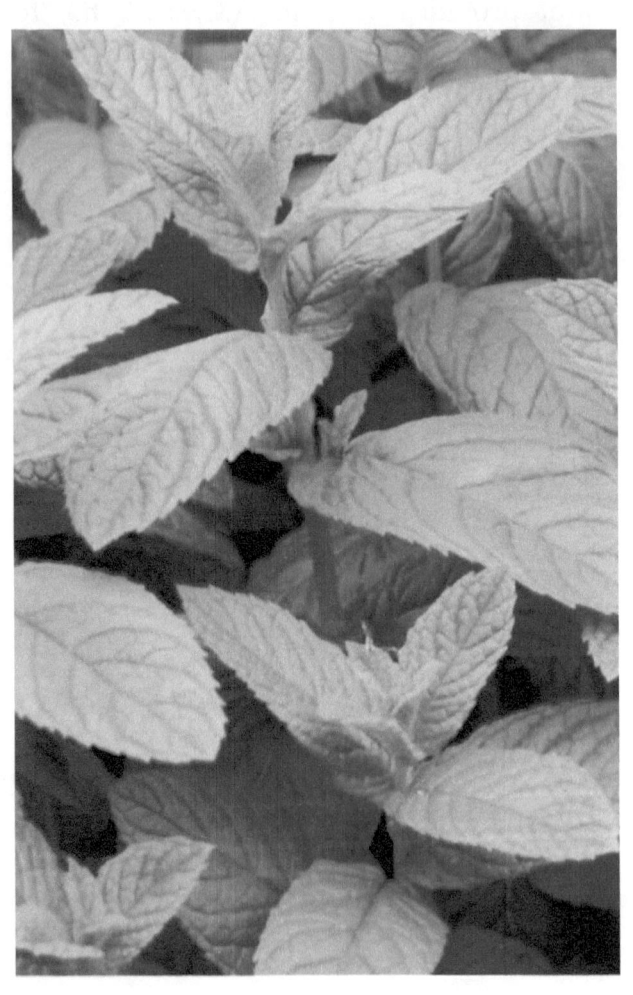

Milk thistle: Silybum marianum

Healing properties:

- antioxidant
- enhances memory
- anti cancer
- protects heart
- boosts weight loss and burning fat
- controls glucose levels
- hepatitis – used to cure ailments of the liver caused by chemotherapy or alcohol
- anti toxic
- lung therapy
- kidney therapy
- prostate problems
- protects heart
- anti diabetes
- spleen anomalies
- pms
- dieuretic

flower can be eaten before blooming and leaves can be eaten when early sprung after cautiously ridding of all thorns, raw or cooked.

Vitamins & minerals : A,C,B,O,calcium, potassium,phosphorous,magnesium and more

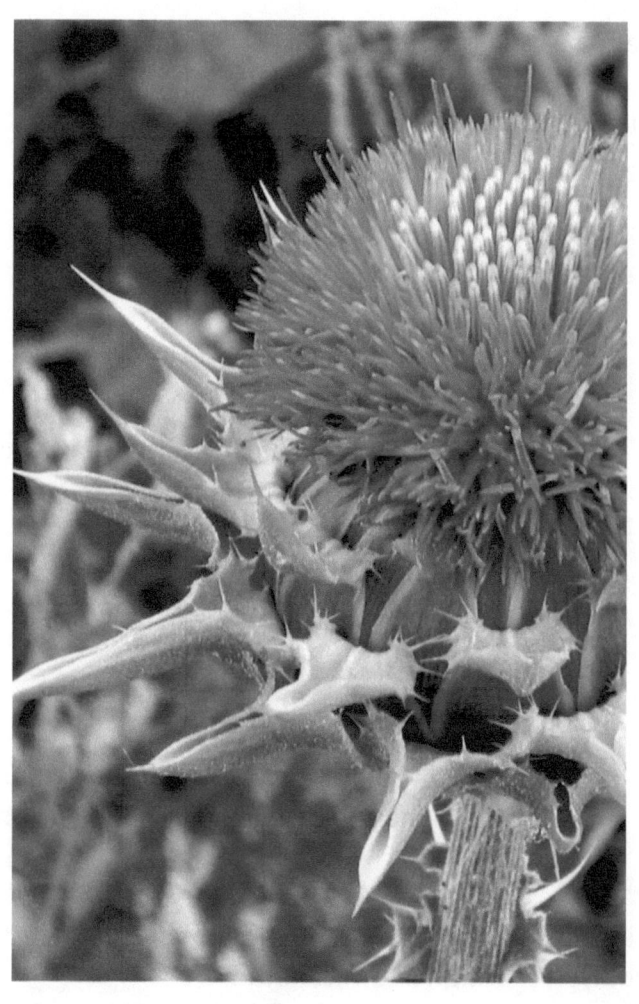

Sage : Salvia officinalis

Healing properties:

- nervous exhaustion
- symtoms of cold and flu
- asthma and cough
- diabetes
- excessive sweat
- diuretic
- natural tonic for healthy face hair and skin
- reduces cellulite
- increases blood circulation
- minimizes and delays wrinkles as it stimulates cell renewal
- gum disease
- mouth sores
- hormonal balance - helps body adjust during menopause minimizing hot flashes

vitamins & minerals: iron, potassium,magnesium,calcium, zinc,manganese,vitamins C,K,A,B, B6 niacin , beta carotene, folic acid, fiber

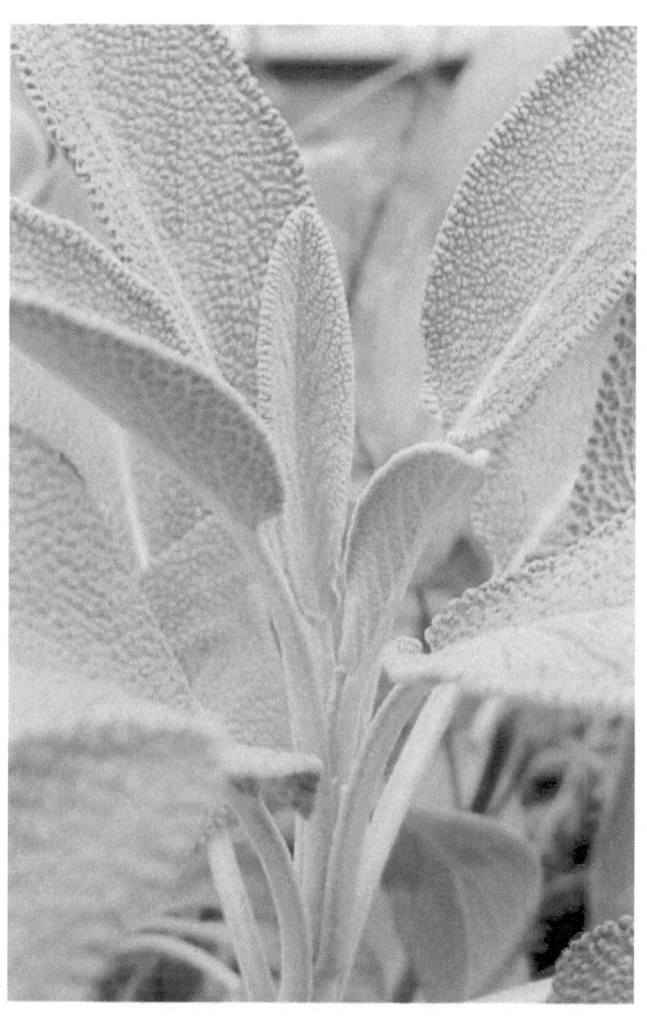

Dittany:Originum dictamnus
(Endangered species)
Used in Minoan Crete

Healing properties:

- Cold and flu symptoms
- Sedative
- Stimulant
- Detoxifier
- Stomach pains
- anemia
- Osteoporosis
- Beneficial for heart blood vessels
- Heals, tones, nourishes
- Hydrates skin
- Anti ageing properties
- Reduces cellulite
- Bad breath
- Anti oxidant
- anti microbe
- anti hemorrhage due to oestrogen action
- anti spasm, naturally heals headaches
- septic
- nerve disordes
- diuretic helps kidneys

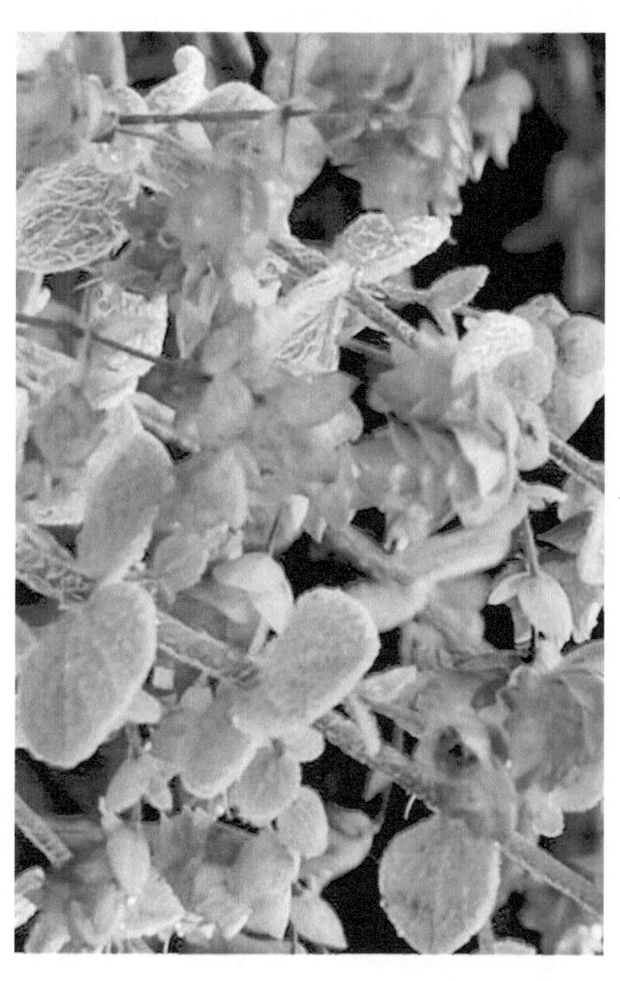

Pennyroyal: wild mint: Mentha pulegium

Healing properties:

tea:
- anti spasm
- stimulant
- diuretic
- helps digestive system
- helps liver
- cleanses gall bladder
- migraines
- bronchitis
- diarrhea

gargle:
- asthma
- flu
- pharyngitis
- laryngitis
- cough

chew leaves:
- Nausea

It can be used for an insect repellant to rid of parasites, ticks and rats.

Rub leaves on mosquito bite to calm the itch

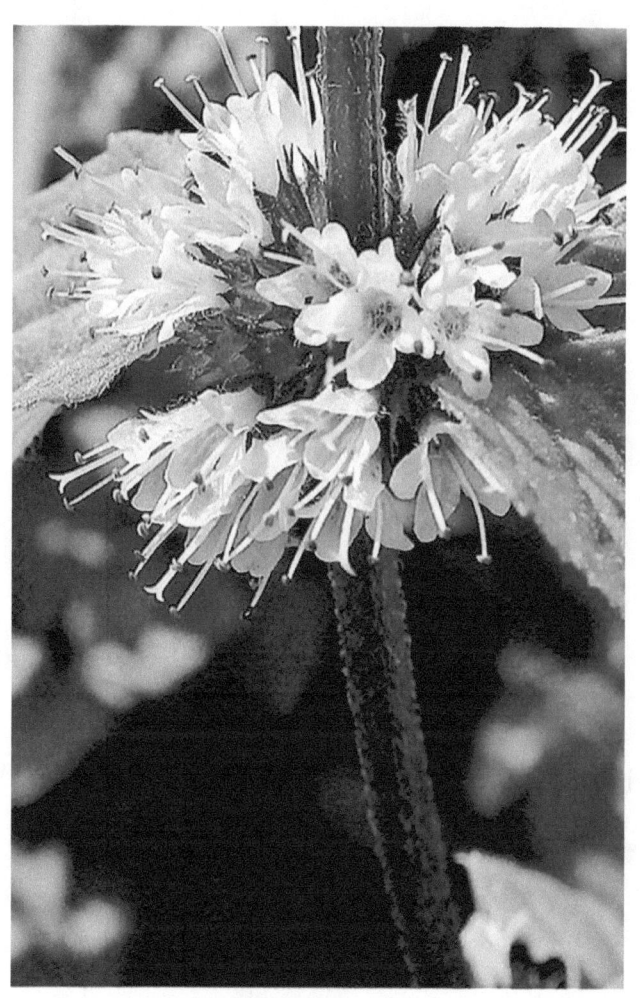

Clalendula:English marigold:Calendula officianalis

Healing properties:

- antiseptic
- acne
- warts
- cuts& wounds
- menstrual regulator
- mosquito bites
- anti flammatory
- antiseptic
- anti hemmerage
- digestion
- cleanses toxins out of the liver and gall bladder

vitamin C, calcium, flavanoids, vitamin A, carotene

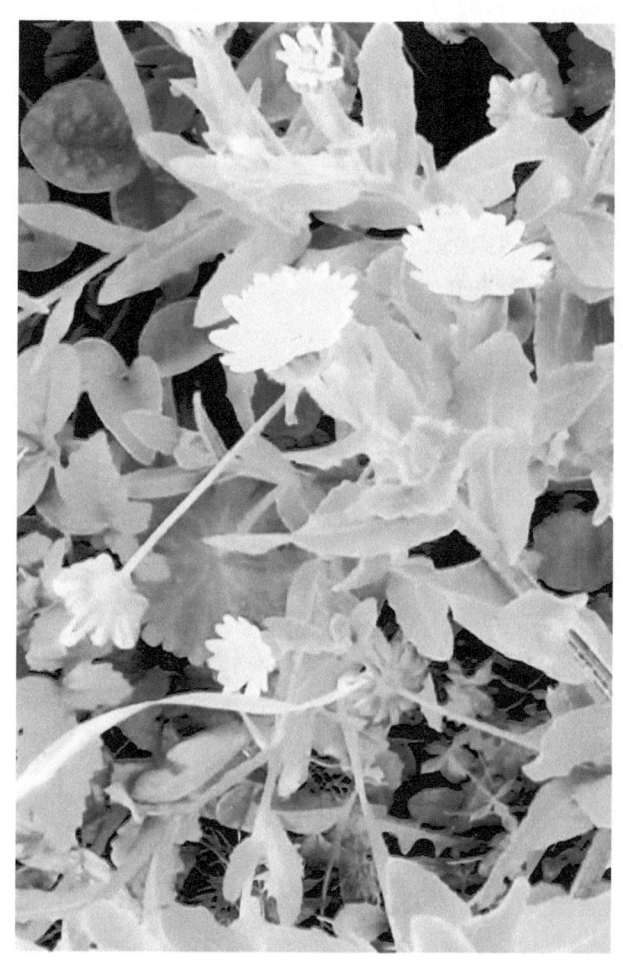

St. John's wort :Hypericum perforatum

Healing properties:

- a natural antidepressant
- stress and anxiety
- anti flammatory
- diuretic
- septic
- menopause symtoms
- stomache ulcers
- bronchitis
- Muscle pians
- Eczema
- Bruises rheumatic pains
- Arthritis
- Burns
- spider veins
- makes scars disappear
- analgesic
- dysentery
- liver problems

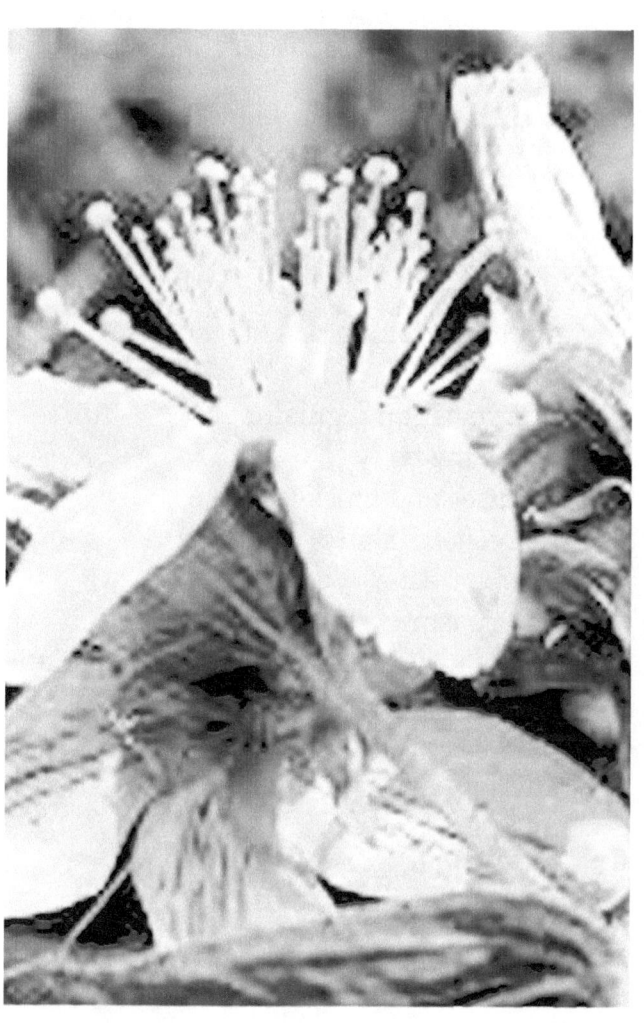

Lemon balm of Crete: Melissa offinalis

Healing properties:

- anxiety
- insomnia
- digestion
- stomach cramps
- fever
- menstruation regulator
- calms the body
- cleanses and tones
- rejuvenates skin
- combats acne
- anti spasm
- stimulates heart and blood circulation thus lowers blood pressure
- natural antihistamine
- allergies and hay fever
- anti bacterial
- fights flu bugs
- herpes and fevers
- helps digestion – used regurlarly protects from stomach ulcers
- anti depressant as it loweres stress and anxiety naturally
- raises perception, boosts memory and helps alzheimers patients
- peridontitis
- intestine parasites

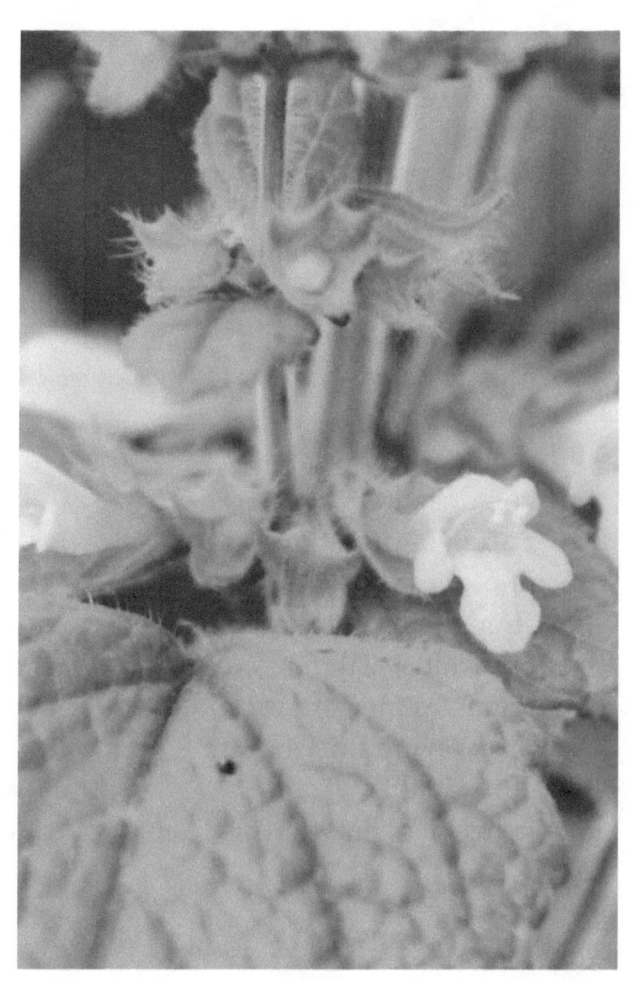

Rosemary:Rosemarinus officinalis

Healing properties:

- boosts blood circulation
- heals wounds
- hair strengthener
- muscle pains
- cold & flu
- rheumatism
- hemorrhoids
- improves digestion
- improves concentration
- strengthens immune system
- bronchitis, asthma
- regulates menstruation
- protects immune system
- antioxidant
- helps in atherosclerosis

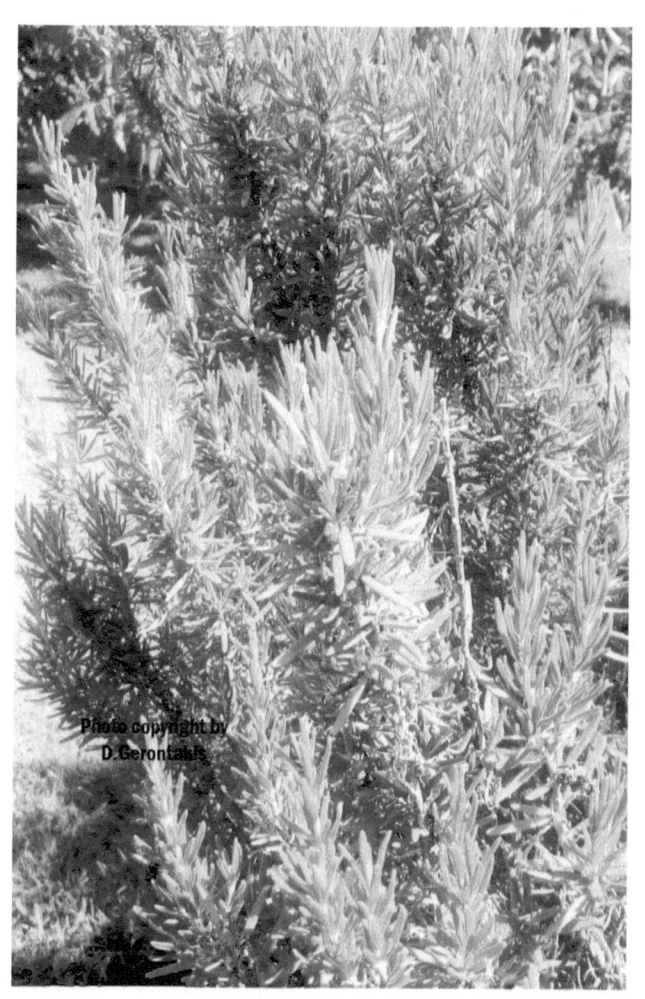

57

Lavender: Lavendula angustifolia

Healing properties:

- anxiety
- sedative and hypnotic
- neurological discomforts
- migraines
- cramps
- rheumatism
- muscle relaxant
- eases tension
- energizes
- cleanses skin
- insomnia
- skin softener

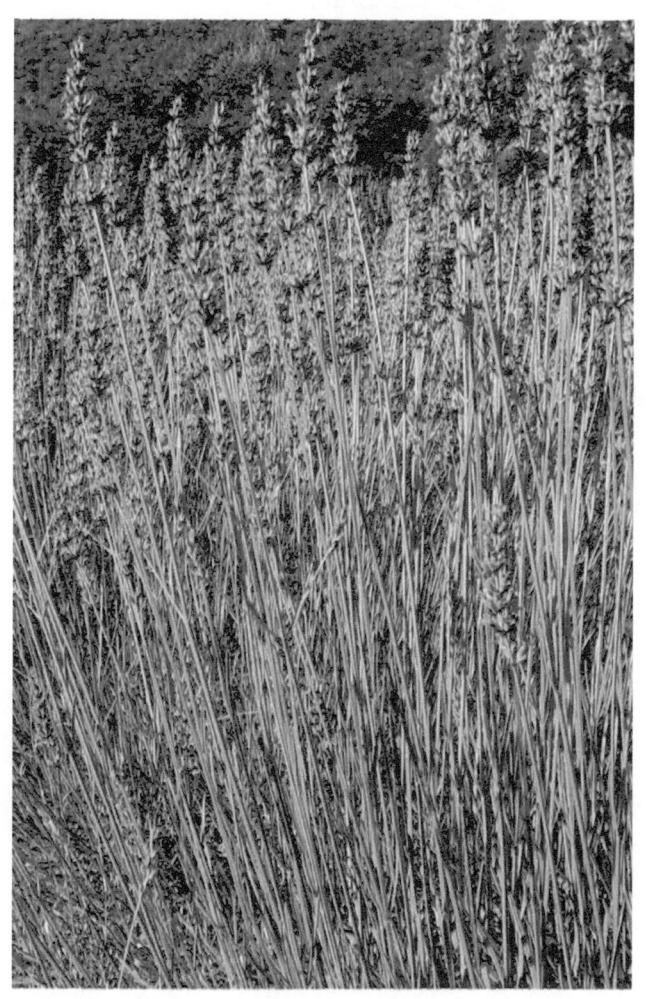

Sheperds tea: Sideritis

Healing properties:

- cold and flu
- respiratory infections
- digestion
- analgesic
- anti spasm
- antioxidant
- anti stress
- works against Alzheimer's disease
- prevents osteoporosis
- anti bacterial
- heal wounds
- enhances heart function
- helps inflammation of the stomach, intestine and urinary tract
- detoxification of the liver and kidneys
- helps anemia as it has plenty of iron
- combats viral infection
- fevers
- high blood pressure
- fights cancer cells

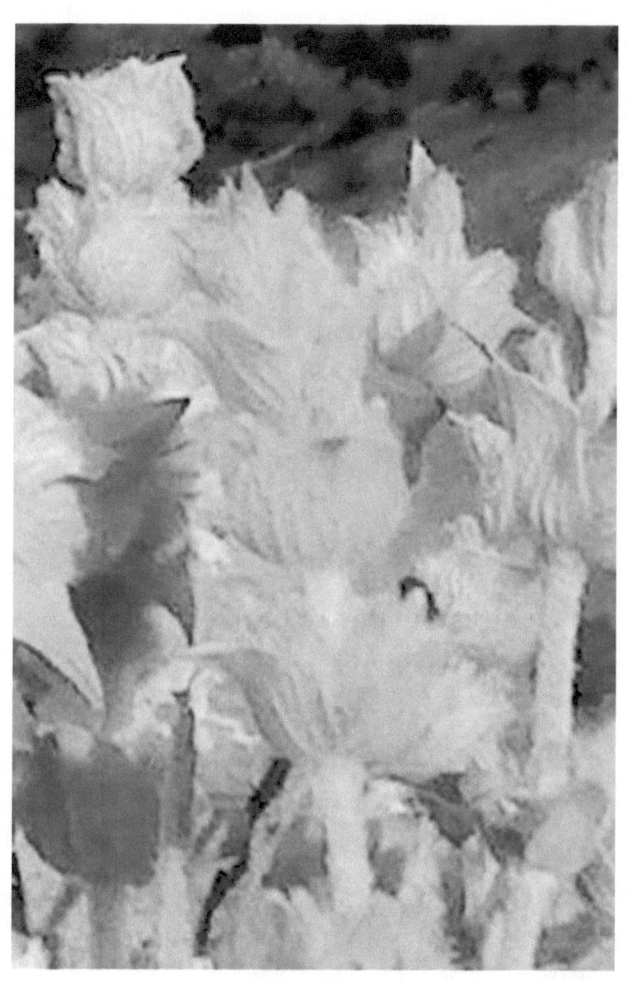

Marathos : Fennel: Foeniculum vulgare

Healing properties:

- boosts lactation
- stomach aches
- eye problems
- gall bladder cleansing
- boosts weight loss
- breaks down fat
- gas reduction
- rheumatism
- muscle spasm
- muscle pain
- reduces inflammation therefore is known to protect against cancer

Vitamins and minerals: A, C, B3, B6, fiber, manganese, potassium, magnesium , iron , calcium,phosperous, zinc, niacin

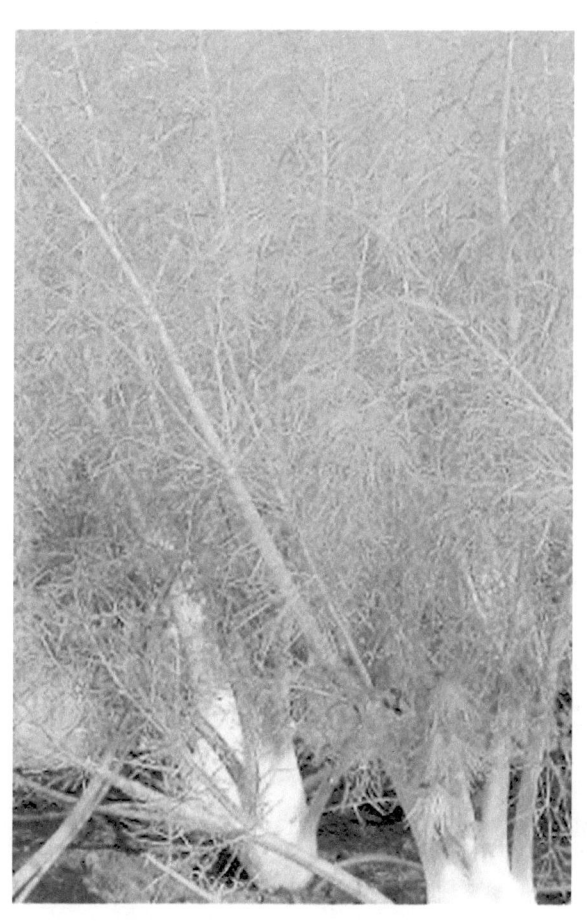

Stamnagathi - Wild Green: Cichorium spinosum

Healing properties:

- cleanses gall bladder
- liver cleanser
- antioxidant
- protects heart
- anti - ageing properties for bone health
- digestion boost
- lowers cholesterol
- diabetes
- aids weight loss
- rheumatism
- reduces bloating during pms
- diuretic

Vitamins and minerals: A, C, E beta carotene, iron potassium phosphorus etc.

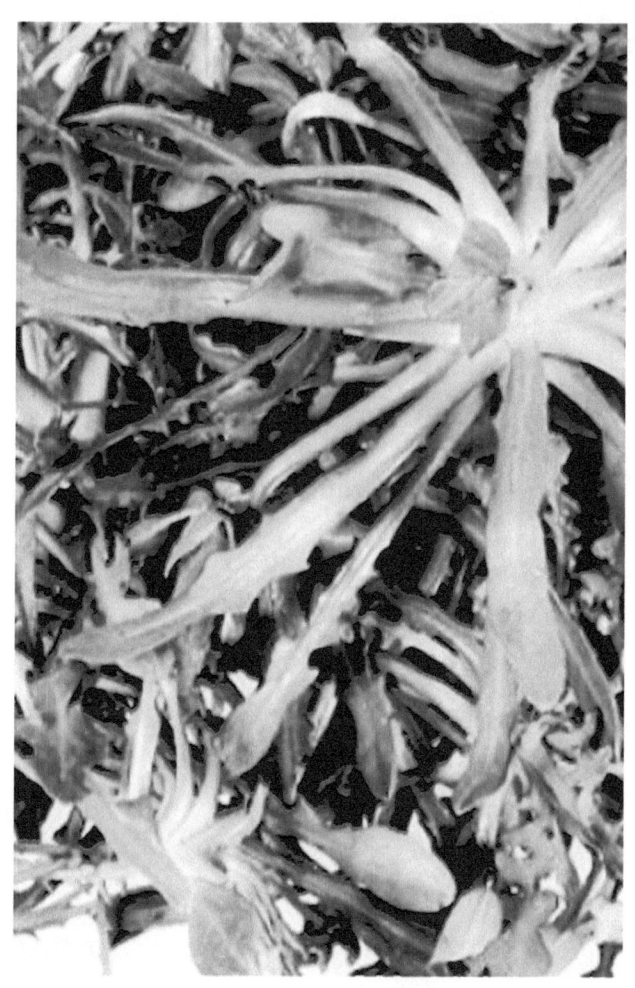

Kalokimithia or Malotira: Sideritis syriaca: the mountain tea of Crete

Healing properties:

- detoxifying,
- anti flammatory
- anti microbial
- antioxidant
- diuretic
- eases stomach ailments
- cough
- cold & flu
- beneficial to blood vessels
- respiratory
- anti ageing properties

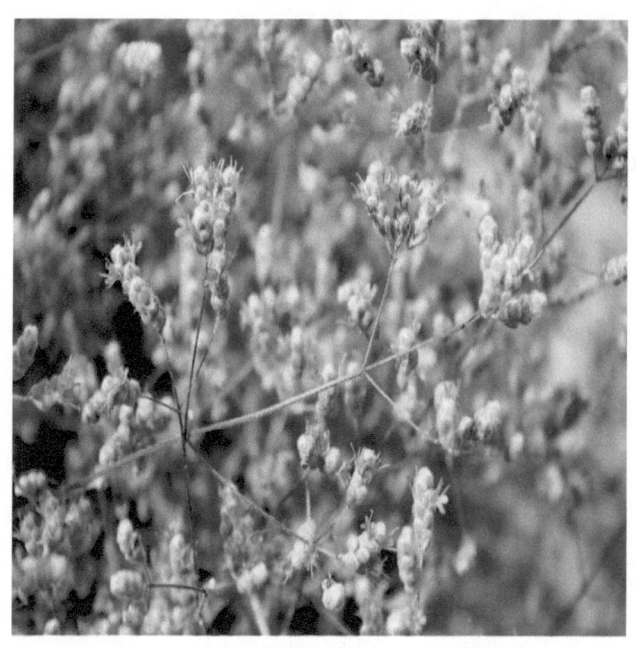

Mullein: Verbascum thaspus

Healing properties:

- diuretic
- mild sedative
- bronchitis
- cold
- cough
- anti - flammatory
- uric acid
- skin irritations
- burns
- eye infections
- diarrhea

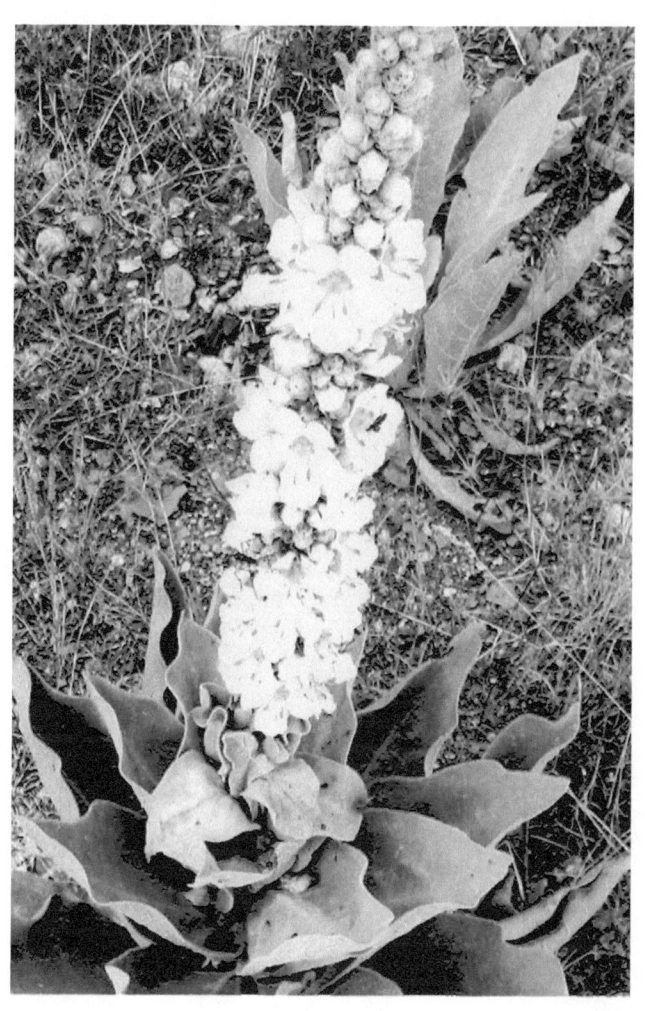